MARY HOPEFIELD

Demystifying the Differences between Anxiety attacks and Panic attacks

Contents

1

Introduction

In a quiet coffee shop nestled within the bustling heart of a city, Sarah sat alone at a table, her hands trembling as she clutched her cup of untouched coffee. The world around her seemed to blur and spin, and the once-familiar sights and sounds now felt alien and threatening. Her heart raced as though it had taken off on a journey of its own, its relentless pounding echoing in her ears. Sarah's palms were slick with sweat, and her chest constricted with a vice-like grip. To any onlooker, she appeared to be a picture of calm; inside, she was trapped in a storm of anxiety and fear.

This is not just Sarah's story; it is the story of countless individuals who grapple with the often silent and invisible battles within their minds. Anxiety and panic attacks, though intangible, are potent adversaries. They can strike suddenly and without warning, leaving those who experience them feeling helpless, lost in the tumultuous sea of their own emotions. It's a universal human experience that transcends borders, cultures, and backgrounds.

This book is about Understanding and hope in the face of these formidable adversaries. Its purpose is to illuminate the complexities of anxiety and panic attacks, revealing the inner workings of the mind and offering a lifeline to those seeking relief and solace. We embark on a journey that blends scientific exploration with the warmth of shared experiences, using real-life anecdotes to illustrate the profound impact of these conditions.

Throughout the chapters that follow, we will delve into the intricate tapestry of anxiety and panic, dissecting the biological, psychological, and emotional elements that interlace to create this very human experience. From the physiological processes within our bodies to the cognitive patterns within our minds, we will seek to demystify these conditions, breaking them down into manageable fragments that can be understood and confronted.

This book is structured with a carefully balanced blend of science and compassion. We will explore the roots of anxiety and panic, the triggers that set them in motion, and the coping strategies that can offer respite. Drawing on scientific explanations and real-life anecdotes, we aim to foster a profound sense of empathy and empowerment for those who face these challenges and those who wish to support them.

In the chapters that follow, we'll navigate the labyrinth of anxiety and panic, providing practical insights, tools, and strategies to manage their impact on our lives. Together, we will learn how to illuminate the shadows of our minds, find our way through the storm, and discover that there is indeed hope for a brighter tomorrow.

As we traverse this terrain, remember that you are not alone. Your struggles, fears, and moments of triumph are mirrored in the experiences of others. Throughout this book, you'll encounter the stories of individuals who have faced anxiety and panic attacks head-on, each narrative a testament to resilience and the human spirit's capacity for healing.

We approach anxiety and panic attacks with a balanced perspective, understanding that they are both deeply rooted in science and profoundly affected by the unique circumstances and emotions of individuals. Our goal is to provide a holistic view, recognizing that while these conditions have biological and neurological components, they also intersect with our thoughts, emotions, and life circumstances.

By the time you reach the final pages of this book, I hope that you will not only understand anxiety and panic attacks more profoundly but also possess a toolbox of strategies for managing and reducing their impact. We offer various coping techniques, from relaxation methods and mindfulness practices to insights into the power of social support and professional help. This book is your guide, your companion on a journey towards greater mental well-being.

Together, we embark on a voyage of Understanding, compassion, and empowerment. We will navigate the challenges posed by anxiety and panic attacks, illuminating the path towards resilience and recovery. The journey may be extended and, at times, arduous, but with knowledge, support, and hope, we are better equipped to find solace and healing in the shadows of our minds.

Welcome to this exploration of the intricate world of anxiety and panic – let's begin the journey.

2

Anxiety and Panic Unveiled

Before we delve into the intricate world of anxiety and panic disorders, let's begin with a few astonishing statistics. In the fast-paced, ever-changing world we inhabit, anxiety and panic are no strangers. They seep into the lives of individuals from all walks of life, silently casting their shadows. It's crucial to comprehend the scale of these challenges:

- **Statistical Revelation 1:** Anxiety disorders are the most common mental health disorders worldwide, affecting an estimated 284 million people, according to the World Health Organization.
- **Statistical Revelation 2:** In the United States alone, panic disorder affects around 6 million adults. These individuals often endure recurrent, unexpected panic attacks, which can be debilitating.
- **Statistical Revelation 3:** Anxiety and panic disorders are not limited by age, and a surprising 10-20% of children and adolescents worldwide experience such conditions.

Now that we've caught your attention with these eye-opening statistics, let's embark on a journey to understand the world of anxiety.

Understanding and Demystifying Anxiety Attacks and Panic Attacks

Clarity and Understanding In mental health, clarity is a precious commodity. It empowers individuals to confront their challenges head-on, fostering a sense of control and Understanding. For anxiety and panic attacks, understanding is not just important; it's essential. Seek straightforward, accessible explanations that demystify these conditions and help them distinguish between them.

Anxiety Attacks

Anxiety is a common emotion that everyone experiences at some point in their lives. It's a natural response to stress or perceived threats. Anxiety attacks, also known as anxiety episodes or flare-ups, are more intense periods of anxiety. They typically have specific triggers, such as a stressful event or situation. These attacks are often characterized by excessive worry, restlessness, and physical symptoms like a racing heart, sweating, and muscle tension. However, it's important to note that anxiety attacks usually build up gradually, giving individuals some time to recognize and manage their symptoms.

Panic Attacks

Panic attacks, on the other hand, are often less predictable and can strike suddenly and without warning. They are intense and overwhelming episodes of fear or terror, and they are not always linked to a specific stressor. Panic attacks can manifest with a wide range of symptoms, including fear of the terrible sensations your body is experiencing, heart palpitations, shortness of breath, trembling, dizziness, and a feeling of impending doom. What sets panic attacks apart is their abrupt onset and their ability to peak within minutes.

Key Differences

- **Onset:** The timing of the start is a critical distinction. Anxiety attacks typically build up gradually and are triggered by a specific source of stress or worry. Panic attacks, in contrast, come on suddenly and often without an apparent trigger.
- **Duration:** Anxiety attacks may last longer, sometimes hours, and can be persistent over several days. Panic attacks, on the other hand, tend to be shorter in duration, usually peaking within minutes and subsiding relatively quickly.
- **Intensity:** Panic attacks are often more intense, featuring overwhelming feelings of terror, whereas anxiety attacks, while distressing, are generally less severe.
- **Specific Triggers:** Anxiety attacks are often linked to identifiable stressors or worries, whereas panic attacks can occur seemingly out of the blue.
- **Recognizability:** Because anxiety attacks build up more gradually, individuals may have a better chance to recognize and manage their symptoms. Panic attacks can be so sudden and severe that they are sometimes mistaken for life-threatening emergencies.

Understanding these distinctions is crucial because the management and treatment approaches for anxiety and panic attacks can differ. While anxiety attacks can often be managed by addressing the underlying stressors and utilizing relaxation techniques, panic attacks may require specialized interventions like cognitive-behavioral therapy and medication.

In conclusion, clarity and Understanding are paramount when dealing with anxiety and panic attacks. By demystifying these conditions and recognizing the key differences, individuals can better identify and manage their symptoms, paving a road for improved mental well-being and a greater sense of control of their lives.

Effective Coping Strategies for Managing Anxiety and Panic Attacks

Anxiety and panic attacks can be incredibly distressing, but the good news is that there are practical techniques and tools to help manage and reduce their impact on your life. If you're seeking actionable advice to alleviate symptoms and improve your mental well-being, you've come to the right place. Here are some effective coping strategies:

1. Deep Breathing and Relaxation Techniques

- Deep breathing exercises can be a lifesaver during the time of an anxiety or panic attack. Try the 4-7-8 technique: Inhale for a count of 4, hold your breath for seven, and exhale for 8. This helps calm your nervous system.
- Practice progressive muscle relaxation by tensing and then releasing each muscle group in your body. This can alleviate physical tension.

2. Mindfulness and Meditation

- Mindfulness techniques, such as meditation and guided meditation, can help you stay grounded and present in the moment. These practices teach you to observe your thoughts without judgment, reducing the impact of anxiety.

3. Cognitive-behavioral therapy (CBT)

- CBT is a practical therapeutic approach for controlling anxiety and panic. It helps you identify and challenge irrational thought patterns, replacing them with more rational, balanced thinking.

4. Lifestyle Modifications

- Regular exercise helps reduce anxiety and panic symptoms. It releases endorphins, the body's natural stress relievers. Implementing a balanced diet and reducing caffeine and sugar intake, as these substances can exacerbate anxiety and panic attacks.
- Ensure you get adequate sleep, as fatigue can increase vulnerability to anxiety.

5. Support System

- Reach out to friends and family for support. Talking about your experiences can help you feel understood and less alone.
- Therapy and counseling can provide valuable tools and strategies for managing anxiety and panic attacks.

6. Medication

- Medication prescribed by a healthcare professional are necessary to manage severe anxiety or panic attacks. These medications can help rebalance brain chemistry and reduce the frequency and intensity of episodes.

7. Self-Care

- Practicing self-care is essential. This includes setting time for activities you enjoy, getting enough rest, and managing stress in your daily life.

8. Identifying Triggers

- Pay attention to what triggers your anxiety or panic attacks. Once you understand the triggers, you can take steps to avoid or cope with them more effectively.

9. Visualization and Affirmations

- Visualize a safe, calming place when you start to feel anxious. Use positive affirmations to counter negative thoughts.

10. Avoidance vs. Exposure

- It's essential to strike a balance between avoiding triggering situations and gradually exposing yourself to them. Gradual exposure can help desensitize your anxiety responses over time.

3

The Healing Power of Spirituality: Overcoming Anxiety and Panic Attacks

In the modern world, we often find ourselves navigating a relentless sea of stress, uncertainties, and challenges. In this turbulent environment, anxiety and panic attacks have become pervasive, affecting millions of lives. Coping with these conditions can be a daunting journey, but many individuals have discovered an unexpected source of strength and solace on their path to healing: spirituality.

- **The Multifaceted Battle Against Anxiety and Panic**

Anxiety and panic attacks are multifaceted adversaries, affecting not only our mental and emotional well-being but also taking a toll on our physical health. The search for coping strategies and relief often leads individuals down numerous paths, including therapy, medication, and lifestyle changes. But for some, there is another dimension to healing – a spiritual one.

- **Connecting with the Inner Self**

Spirituality, in this context, is not limited to any specific religion or belief system. It encompasses a deep connection with one's inner self and a profound understanding of the greater universe. It involves cultivating a sense of purpose and meaning in life, which can be a powerful force against the overwhelming waves of anxiety and panic.

• The Importance of Faith

Spirituality often involves faith, whether in a higher power, the interconnectedness of all living things, or the potential for personal growth. This faith can serve as an anchor during tumultuous times, offering a sense of security and purpose that can counteract the fear and uncertainty that often accompany anxiety and panic attacks.

• Mindfulness and Meditation

Many spiritual practices include mindfulness and meditation, which are powerful tools for managing anxiety and panic. These techniques encourage individuals to focus on the present moment, cultivating an awareness of their thoughts and emotions. By learning to observe their internal experiences without judgment, individuals can gain greater control over their responses to anxiety triggers.

• Strengthening Resilience

Spirituality often emphasizes resilience, teaching individuals to endure adversity and emerge stronger. This quality is invaluable when facing the challenges of anxiety and panic. By drawing on their spiritual beliefs, individuals can find the inner strength to weather the storms and persist in their journey toward healing.

- ## The Sense of Community

Another vital aspect of spirituality is the sense of community. Whether through a religious congregation, meditation group, or simply connecting with like-minded individuals, the support of a community can be a tremendous source of comfort and Understanding. Sharing one's experiences and receiving support from others who have faced similar challenges can be profoundly healing.

- ## Empowering Hope

In the face of anxiety and panic, spirituality offers a beacon of hope. It encourages individuals to believe in the possibility of recovery, the potential for growth, and the capacity for personal transformation. This hope can be a powerful motivator, inspiring individuals to take the necessary steps toward healing.

While spirituality is not a one-size-fits-all solution, it has provided solace and strength to many who confront anxiety and panic attacks. Its role is not to replace traditional treatment methods but to complement them, offering a holistic approach to healing. By acknowledging the importance of the spiritual dimension in the journey toward recovery, individuals can find the inner resources to overcome their challenges and build a brighter future.

Remember that coping strategies vary from person to person, and what works best for you may differ from what works for someone else. Experiment with different techniques and find what resonates with you. Additionally, be patient with yourself – managing anxiety and panic attacks is a journey, and it's okay to seek professional help if you're struggling.

Effective coping strategies are essential for managing anxiety and panic attacks. Incorporating these techniques into your daily life and seeking support can reduce the impact of these conditions, alleviate symptoms, and improve your overall mental well-being.

It's important to remember that managing anxiety and panic attacks is a process, and there may be setbacks along the way. However, by implementing these coping strategies and seeking support, individuals can take control of their symptoms and work towards improved mental health. Don't hesitate to reach out for help if needed, and remember that you are not alone in your journey toward healing.

4

Empathy and Support for Those Dealing with Anxiety and Panic Attacks

Dealing with anxiety and panic attacks is an isolating and overwhelming experience. Many individuals facing these issues seek a sense of community and Reassurance. They want to know they are not alone in their struggles and that there is hope for a brighter future. Here's how to provide empathy and support to those in need:

1. Be a Good Listener

One of the most potent ways to support someone with anxiety or panic attacks is to be there and listen. Create a safe space to express their feelings and experiences without judgment. Oftentimes, just having someone to talk to can be immensely Comforting.

2. Educate Yourself

Take the time to educate yourself about anxiety and panic attacks. Understanding the conditions, their symptoms, and common triggers will help you empathize with the person dealing with them. Knowledge can also help you offer better support.

3. Offer Reassurance

Let the individual know that their feelings are valid and that you care about their well-being. Reassure them that you are there to support them through the challenges they face.

4. Avoid Minimizing or Dismissing Their Feelings

Avoid saying things like "calm down" or "it's not a big deal." Such statements can make the person feel unheard or invalidated. Instead, acknowledge their feelings and encourage them to express themselves.

5. Encourage Professional Help

If the anxiety or panic attacks are severe or persistent, encourage the person to seek professional help. Therapists, counselors, and medical professionals can provide specialized support and treatment options.

6. Be Patient

Recovery from anxiety and panic attacks is not always linear. There will be ups and downs along the way. Patience and Understanding are crucial as the individual navigates their path to healing.

7. Respect Boundaries

Respect the individual's boundaries and comfort levels. Some people may want more support and involvement, while others may need space.

Please ask them what they need and be willing to adjust your approach accordingly.

8. Share Resources

Please provide them with information about support groups, helplines, or books that can be beneficial. Knowing that resources are available can offer a sense of hope and empowerment.

9. Encourage Self-Care

Emphasize the importance of self-care. Encourage the person to look into activities that promote relaxation and well-being, such as exercise, meditation, or hobbies they enjoy.

10. Stay Connected

Continue to check in and maintain contact. Isolation can exacerbate anxiety and panic attacks, so staying connected and showing that you care is invaluable.

11. Share Stories of Hope

Share stories of people who have successfully managed their anxiety or panic attacks. Knowing that others have overcome similar challenges can provide hope and inspiration.

12. Be Non-Judgmental

Avoid passing judgment or offering unsolicited advice. Remember that each person's experience is unique, and what works for one may not work for another.

Empathy and support are essential for those dealing with anxiety and panic attacks. By creating a caring, non-judgmental, and understanding environment, you can help individuals feel less alone and give them the hope they need to envision a brighter future. Your support can make a significant difference in their journey toward better mental health.

Remember that dealing with anxiety and panic attacks can be a long and challenging journey. It is essential to be patient and Understanding, as recovery takes time. Celebrate their successes, no matter how small, and remind them that setbacks are a natural part of the process. Keep in mind that supporting someone through anxiety and panic attacks can be emotionally taxing, so be sure to prioritize your self-care as well. By working together and fostering a supportive community, we can help individuals facing these challenges feel heard, validated, and hopeful.

5

What is Anxiety?

Anxiety is a universal human emotion. It's the quiet tremor in your chest before a big presentation, the fluttering in your stomach on a first date, or the cautious excitement as you board an airplane to a far-off destination. In its essence, anxiety is the body's natural response to perceived threats or stressors.

At its core, anxiety prepares us to face challenges, whether they are real or imagined. It's the evolutionary hand-me-down that once helped our ancestors escape predators, find food, and protect their kin. This response is hardwired into our biology and psychology and continues to serve a vital function in our lives.

Common Symptoms of Anxiety

Understanding anxiety also means recognizing its various manifestations. Anxiety can manifest in many ways, and its symptoms are as diverse as the people who experience it. Common symptoms include:

- **Physical Symptoms:** Rapid heartbeat, shallow breathing, muscle tension, sweating, and stomach discomfort.

- **Cognitive Symptoms:** Excessive worry, racing thoughts, an inability to concentrate, and catastrophic thinking.
- **Emotional Symptoms:** Irritability, restlessness, a sense of impending doom, and a feeling of being on edge.
- **Behavioral Symptoms:** Avoidance of triggers or situations, seeking Reassurance, and physical rituals, like tapping or checking.

Causes of Anxiety

Anxiety doesn't emerge from thin air. Various factors contribute to its development, and it's often a complex interplay of these factors. Some common causes of anxiety include:

- **Biological Factors:** Genetics can play a significant role. If anxiety disorders run in the family, there may be a genetic predisposition. Additionally, imbalances in neurotransmitters, such as serotonin, can contribute to anxiety.
- **Environmental Factors:** Traumatic life events, such as accidents, abuse, or loss, can trigger anxiety. Chronic stress, ongoing exposure to stressful environments, or a lack of social support can also increase vulnerability.
- **Psychological Factors:** Personality traits, like perfectionism or a tendency to catastrophize, can make individuals more prone to anxiety. Childhood experiences and learned behaviors may also contribute.

It's important to note that anxiety is an ordinary and necessary part of life. However, in some cases, it can become overwhelming and interfere with daily activities. When anxiety becomes chronic and excessive, it can lead to an anxiety disorder. It affects millions of people each year. Some common anxiety disorders include obsessive-compulsive disorder., generalized anxiety disorder, panic disorder, and social anxiety disorder. Managing anxiety can be a complex process, and there is no one-size-fits-all solution. However, several strategies can help individuals cope with anxiety, including therapy, medication, and lifestyle changes. It's also essential to seek support from loved ones and mental health professionals. With the right tools and resources, it is possible to manage anxiety and lead a fulfilling life.

6

What is a Panic Attack?

While anxiety is the whisper of worry, a panic attack is a sudden, intense scream of fear and death. It's a storm that brews in the blink of an eye, overwhelming the body and the mind. So, what exactly is a panic attack?

A panic attack is a short but intense rise of overwhelming fear or distress. A sudden and unexpected onset of severe physical and psychological symptoms characterizes it. These symptoms can include shortness of breath, racing heart, chest pain, trembling, dizziness, and a feeling of impending doom. It's as if the body's alarm system has gone haywire, initiating a "fight or flight" response when there is no apparent danger.

Recognizing Panic Attack Symptoms

The symptoms of a panic attack are both diverse and debilitating. Here are some common manifestations to watch out for:

- **Rapid Heartbeat:** The heart races as if it's in a race against time.
- **Shortness of Breath:** Breathing becomes shallow and fast, leaving

the individual gasping for air.

- **Chest Pain:** A crushing or squeezing sensation in the chest is common and often mistaken for a heart attack.
- **Trembling and Shaking:** The body may tremble uncontrollably.
- **Dizziness:** Vertigo and a spinning sensation can be overwhelming.
- **Nausea:** Many individuals experience stomach discomfort and may feel like they're going to be sick, vomit, diarrhea.
- **Chills or Hot Flashes:** The body's temperature regulation goes haywire, leading to alternating sensations of cold and heat.
- **Feelings of Unreality:** Detachment from reality or feeling like the world isn't real.

Triggers of Panic Attacks

Panic attacks, like anxiety, don't occur in a vacuum. They often have identifiable triggers, varying significantly from person to person. Some common triggers include:

- **Stress:** High-stress situations, such as work deadlines, relationship problems, or financial concerns, can provoke panic attacks.
- **Phobias:** enclosed spaces; specific phobias, such as fear of heights or public speaking, can trigger panic attacks when confronted with the feared situation.
- **Trauma:** Past traumatic experiences can lead to panic attacks, especially if these experiences are reminiscent of the original trauma.
- **Medical Conditions:** Some medical conditions, like hyperthyroidism, can cause panic-like symptoms.
- **Caffeine or Stimulants:** Consumption of caffeine, certain medications, or recreational drugs can provoke panic attacks.

John's Struggle with Anxiety and Panic

To truly understand the impact of anxiety and panic attacks, let's delve into the life of John, a person who grapples with both conditions. John's journey is a testament to the challenges and triumphs that individuals with these conditions face daily.

A Storm Within John's Story

John is an ordinary man living an extraordinary life. He's a dedicated father, a loving husband, and a successful IT manager at a large corporation. Yet, behind the facade of normalcy, John fights a silent battle that many are unaware of.

In his early thirties, John experienced his first panic attack. It struck without warning during a work meeting and felt like a heart attack. The intense chest pain, racing heart, and dizziness left him terrified and confused. Panic attacks would become his uninvited companions, often striking during what should be joyful moments in life.

As we follow John's journey, we will explore the heart-wrenching moments when anxiety and panic threaten to drown him in a sea of fear. We will also witness his remarkable resilience and strategies to navigate the storms within his mind.

John's story serves as a window into the lived experiences of those grappling with anxiety and panic attacks. It's a narrative of hope, courage, and the quest for a brighter tomorrow.

A life with anxiety and panic attacks is a challenging and exhausting experience. The fear and uncertainty that come with these conditions can feel overwhelming and isolating. However, it's crucial to remember that you're not alone. Millions of people worldwide struggle with anxiety and panic attacks, and there are effective treatments available to help manage symptoms.

One of the most crucial steps in managing anxiety and panic attacks is recognizing the symptoms and triggers. By understanding the warning signs, you can take action to reduce the severity of an episode. Additionally, seeking support from friends, family, or a mental health professional can provide unique guidance and assistance.

Remember, healing from anxiety and panic attacks is a journey, and it takes time and effort. But with the proper support and tools, it's possible to overcome the challenges and live a fulfilling life.

7

The Fine Line Between Anxiety and Panic Attacks

Picture anxiety and panic as neighboring houses on a quiet street. They share a white picket fence, their gardens abloom with vibrant emotions. Anxiety resides in the cozy living room, while panic resides in the attic, hidden away but never truly gone. The fence that separates them is the fine line that we must walk, the line that divides the two, sometimes blurring into obscurity.

In this chapter, we'll embark on a journey to spot the subtle distinctions between anxiety and panic. Just like the picket fence, we'll take a closer look at the boundaries that distinguish these experiences from one another, drawing from personal stories and offering practical coping strategies.

Critical Differences Between Anxiety and Panic Attacks

Duration and Intensity

Anxiety often feels like a slow burn. It's the ever-present hum of worry in the background of our lives, varying in intensity but rarely reaching a fever pitch. It can linger for hours, days, or even weeks. Panic, on the other hand, is a sudden blaze, an intense eruption that peaks within minutes. The duration and intensity are key differentiators between these experiences.

Triggers and Anticipation

Anxiety typically has identifiable triggers—a looming work deadline, a social event, or an upcoming exam. While these triggers may induce apprehension, individuals with anxiety can often anticipate and prepare for them. Panic attacks, however, are the unwelcome guests that arrive unannounced. They strike without warning, making anticipation impossible and catching the individual off guard.

Physical Symptoms

The physical symptoms are another area of distinction. Anxiety may manifest with physical symptoms such as muscle tension, restlessness, and a racing heart. While distressing, these symptoms are less severe. In contrast, panic attacks bring a cascade of alarming physical sensations, including chest pain, shortness of breath, and a sense of imminent doom. The intensity and abruptness of these symptoms set panic apart.

Personal Stories: Real-Life Accounts

The Multifaceted Array of Experiences Anxiety and panic attacks are experienced uniquely by each individual. To illustrate this diversity, let's delve into the stories of three individuals who have faced both attacks. Their experiences showcase the intricate tapestry of emotions and responses to anxiety and panic.

- Maria's Struggle: Maria, a university student, describes the relentless grip of anxiety that accompanies her daily life. For her, anxiety was like a constant companion, whispering self-doubt and worry. She shares her journey of recognizing the triggers and seeking therapy to manage her anxiety.
- Alex's Unexpected Panic: Alex, a dedicated teacher, recounts the day he experienced his first panic attack during a staff meeting. The intense physical sensations, which felt like a heart attack, left him stunned. Alex takes us through the challenges he faced in identifying the source of his panic and the steps he took to manage it.
- Emily's Tale of Resilience: Emily, a working mother, shares her experiences with both anxiety and panic attacks. She describes how the two often intertwine, with anxiety acting as a precursor to panic. Emily's story demonstrates the courage and resilience required to navigate the complex landscape of these conditions.

These stories emphasize that the line between anxiety and panic is not a stark divide; it's a blurred frontier, and each person's journey is unique.

Coping Strategies for Each

Breathing Exercises and Relaxation Technique

Both anxiety and panic attacks can benefit from relaxation techniques. Breathing exercises, such as diaphragmatic exercises, can help alleviate symptoms. Learning to relax the body and calm the mind is a valuable tool for both conditions.

Medication and Therapy Options

In cases where symptoms become unmanageable, seeking professional help is crucial. Medications and therapy, particularly cognitive-behavioral therapy (CBT), have proven effective in managing both anxiety and panic disorders. We'll delve deeper into these treatment options.

Lifestyle Changes for Long-Term Management

Long-term management is a critical aspect of coping with anxiety and panic attacks. We'll explore lifestyle changes, such as exercise, nutrition, and stress management, that can reduce the frequency and intensity of these experiences.

By the end of this chapter, you'll have a clearer understanding of the differences between anxiety and panic, and you'll be armed with practical strategies for managing both. The stories of Maria, Alex, and Emily will serve as a reminder that these challenges are part of the human experience, and with knowledge and resilience, they can be conquered.

Shocking Facts about Mental Health Stigma

Despite the prevalence of mental health disorders, studies reveal that nearly two-thirds of people with anxiety and panic attacks never seek treatment. The reason? Stigma. It's a formidable barrier that prevents individuals from seeking the help they need, and it's high time we shatter this barrier.

The stigma surrounding mental health disorders is a pervasive problem. It can take many forms, from the fear of being labeled as "crazy" to the belief that seeking help is a sign or definition of weakness. These attitudes can prevent individuals from seeking the treatment they need, leading to unnecessary suffering and worsening of symptoms.

The facts surrounding mental health stigma are shocking. According to studies, nearly two-thirds of people with anxiety and panic attacks never seek treatment. Many individuals who do seek help face discrimination and negative attitudes from friends, family, and even healthcare providers.

It's time to shatter the stigma surrounding mental health disorders. Education and awareness are critical in breaking down these barriers. By understanding the realities of anxiety and panic attacks, we can eliminate the myths and misconceptions that contribute to stigma.

It's also essential to prioritize mental health care and ensure that everyone has access to the resources they need. This includes destigmatizing mental health treatment and making it readily available and affordable for all.

Breaking the stigma surrounding mental health disorders is a collective effort. By speaking out, supporting those who are struggling, and advocating for change, we can create a world where seeking help for mental health concerns is not only accepted but encouraged.

8

Exploring the Stigma Around Anxiety and Panic Attacks

Historical Perspectives on Mental Health

The stigma surrounding mental health has deep historical roots. For centuries, conditions like anxiety and panic attacks were often misunderstood and attributed to supernatural causes. We'll embark on a journey through time, exploring how society's perceptions of these conditions have evolved and yet how lingering misconceptions persist.

The Impact of Stigma on Individuals

The weight of stigma is not easily shrugged off. It casts shadows that extend beyond the individual's mental health, affecting their self-esteem, relationships, and overall quality of life. We'll delve into the profound impact that stigma has on those living with anxiety and panic attacks, exposing the injustices they face daily.

Success Stories: Inspiring Narratives / Shattering the Chains of

Stigma

In this section, we'll encounter the stories of individuals who have defied stigma and emerged as beacons of hope. These stories illustrate that living with anxiety and panic attacks is not a life sentence and that individuals can thrive despite the challenges they face.

- Ella's Triumph: Ella, a talented artist, will take us on her journey of reclaiming her life from anxiety and panic. Her story is a testament to the transformative power of resilience and self-acceptance.
- James's Resilience: James, a high-achieving executive, shares his experiences breaking free from the stigma associated with mental health disorders. His story showcases the resilience and strength that reside within us all.
- Lena's Advocacy: Lena, a passionate mental health advocate, reflects on her advocacy journey and how she has channeled her own experiences with anxiety into a powerful force for change. Her story demonstrates that confronting stigma head-on can catalyze societal transformation.

Furthermore, this passage on mental health highlights the importance of breaking the chains of stigma. Through success stories and inspiring narratives, we can see that living with anxiety and panic attacks isn't a life sentence. Instead, individuals can thrive despite the challenges they face. The section titled "Shattering the Chains of Stigma" shares the stories of Ella, James, and Lena, who have defied stigma and emerged as beacons of hope.

Ella, a talented artist, showcases the transformative power of resilience and self-acceptance. James, a high-achieving executive, showcases the stability and strength that resides within us all. Lena, a passionate mental health advocate, reflects on her advocacy journey and how she has channeled her own experiences with anxiety into a powerful force for change. Her story shows that confronting stigma head-on can catalyze societal transformation.

It's essential to remark on the stigma surrounding mental health disorders, as it can cast shadows that affect an individual's self-esteem, relationships, and quality of life.

9

Advocating for Mental Health Awareness

In this section, we'll explore practical strategies to combat the stigma surrounding anxiety and panic attacks. These strategies not only empower individuals to seek help but also encourage society to embrace a more inclusive and compassionate perspective.

- **Education and Awareness:** The first step in combating stigma is education. We'll explore how awareness campaigns and mental health education programs can make a significant difference.
- **Challenging Stereotypes:** Challenging stereotypes and dispelling myths is a powerful way to reduce stigma. We'll delve into strategies for altering society's misconceptions about mental health.
- **Advocacy and Support:** Advocacy efforts at the individual and community levels are crucial. We'll discuss how individuals can become advocates for mental health awareness and support those in need.

This chapter is a call to action. It's an invitation to recognize the profound impact of stigma, acknowledge the inspiring narratives of those who have triumphed, and equip ourselves with strategies to break the chains that have held back progress in mental health awareness and support.

The stigma surrounding anxiety and panic attacks can be a huge barrier to those seeking help. Individuals feel ashamed, embarrassed, and frustrated, resulting in people avoiding treatment. However, practical strategies can be employed to combat this stigma, benefiting both individuals and society.

Education and awareness campaigns are essential first steps. By educating people on the nature of anxiety and panic attacks, we can reduce misconceptions and increase Understanding. Mental health education programs can provide tools to help individuals manage their symptoms and encourage them to seek help when needed.

Challenging stereotypes and dispelling myths is another way to combat stigma. This can be achieved by normalizing discussions around mental health, especially in the workplace. By creating a safe place for employees to talk about their mental health, we can reduce the stigma associated with it.

Finally, advocacy and support at the individual and community levels are crucial. Individuals can become advocates for mental health awareness by sharing their stories and experiences. Communities can also support those in need by providing resources and services to help manage anxiety and panic attacks.

It is time to break the chains of stigma surrounding anxiety and panic attacks. By educating ourselves, challenging stereotypes, and advocating for support, we can create a more inclusive and compassionate society. Let us answer the call to action and make a positive change in mental health awareness and support.

10

Conclusion

We've just wrapped up a wild expedition through the intricate jungle of anxiety and panic attacks. We've peeled back the layers of our minds, uncovering the subtle differences between these sneaky foes. We've learned to wrangle these emotions with coping tools ranging from mindfulness to medication. And, if the journey ever gets too rough, we've discovered the power of therapists and the strength of our loved ones.

Now, as we bid farewell to our adventure, let us leave with a message of hope and a hearty dose of resilience. Anxiety and panic attacks are no picnic, but they don't have to rule our lives. We've met some fantastic folks who have faced these challenges head-on, proving that the human spirit is more potent than any shadow. So, my friend, you're not alone in this fight. You've got a tribe of warriors beside you, ready to weather any storm.

Your journey may twist and turn, but you are equipped with the tools to emerge stronger and brighter than before. Don't let anxiety or panic attacks define you. You are defined by your courage and strength. So rise and embrace your journey, for it is a testament to the power of the human spirit.

Anxiety and panic attacks are common health issues that affect millions of people worldwide. Various factors, including stress, trauma, and genetics, can trigger these conditions, which can cause various internal and physical symptoms, such as tachycardia, shortness of breath, sweating, and fear of losing control.

However, as the passage mentions, there are ways to manage these conditions and live a fulfilling life. Coping tools like mindfulness, therapy, and medication can help individuals navigate the challenges of anxiety and panic attacks. Additionally, having a support system for loved ones and fellow warriors can provide a sense of community and strength.

It's important to remember that recovery is not linear, and setbacks may occur. But with resilience and determination, it's possible to overcome these obstacles and emerge stronger than before. Don't let anxiety or panic attacks define you. Your courage and strength define you. So embrace your journey, knowing that you have the power to overcome any challenge that comes your way.

If you are suffering from anxiety or panic attacks, it's essential to prioritize your mental health and seek professional help. A licensed therapist or counselor can provide specialized treatment and support to help you manage your symptoms. Additionally, incorporating self-care practices like exercise, healthy eating, and other great ideas are hobbies that can help reduce stress and improve your overall well-being.

Remember that everyone's experience with anxiety and panic attacks is unique, and there is no one-size-fits-all solution. Don't be afraid to try different strategies and approaches until you find what works for you. With time, patience, and perseverance.

11

Resources

Post | Welllifecounseling. (n.d.). Welllifecounseling. https://www.welllife
counseling.com/post/tips-to-manage-anxiety-on-your-own%20How
%20To%20Respond%20To%20Someone%20With%20Anxiety%20-%2
0AnxietyProHelp.com

O, D. (2022, June 26). How To Respond To Someone With Anxiety -
AnxietyProHelp.com. *AnxietyProHelp.com.* https://www.anxietyprohel
p.com/how-to-respond-to-someone-with-anxiety/

Addicted to Self Help. (n.d.). *stress management Archives - Addicted to Self
Help.* https://addictedtoselfhelp.com/tag/stress-management/

Hypnosis For Anxiety | Albuquerque, NM. (n.d.). Nmhypnosis. https://w
ww.nmhypnosis.com/hypnosis-for-anxiety

Saprea. (2023, September 25). *Anxiety | Saprea.* https://youniquefound
ation.org/resources-for-child-sexual-abuse-survivors/common-symp
toms/stopping-the-cycle-of-anxiety/

Brouillette, J., Cyr, S., Painchaud-Bouchard, A., Marcil, M., & Rhainds, D. (2019). Increased Risk of Coronary Heart Disease in Patients with Anxiety Disorders: A Review of Underlying Biomarkers. *Biomedical Journal of Scientific and Technical Research.* https://doi.org/10.26717/bjs tr.2019.23.003844